50 TOP PALEO RECIPES

Quick and Easy Paleo Diet Recipes for Weight Loss and Optimum Health

EMMA GREEN

Book

4

CONTENTS

FOREWORD

"I love everything about Emma's connection to weight loss and health."

> Hi, my name is Nat Lee, and I've spent most of my life looking
> pretty good and feeling great. That was up until I started
> eating on the run and allowing my busy life as a mom to
> take hold of me. While working too.

> In truth, I knew I should eat great food, but time constraints
> and "motherly craziness" got the better of me. I made sure
> my son ate well. But I didn't, which was silly, really.
> Parenting is one of those things that just takes over your life,
> I suppose. So, anyway, I kinda ate loads of stuff I shouldn't,
> and drank sodas and milkshakes an awful lot. Chocolate
> and takeout became my best friend, and I became
> overweight, by anyone's standards. No one really told me I
> looked bad, I mean, most people aren't that obvious. But
> when I was diagnosed with a severe illness and bedridden

for four years, it became time to do something to help my recovery. I made the change as soon as I could.

Since reading Emma's books, I've lost 18.5 kg (which is 40 amazing pounds). And I've managed to keep it off by following her wonderful advice, and by using her awesome, easy-to-do recipes. I live relatively simply, but her guide to nutrition and her tips and tricks have helped me a bucket load. Thank you Emma, you've literally changed my life!

INTRODUCTION

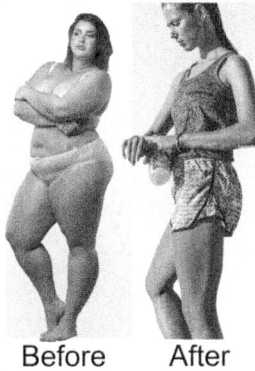

Before   After

Hi! Thanks so much for joining me here. I want to extend a huge, warm welcome to you for taking weight loss or general optimal health into your own hands. I am so excited to share this time with you, and to tell you about my 50 top favorite recipes; the ones that I have managed to get my hands on – and work! Awesome, huh?

I grew up with the Southern style of eating. It was something our family did well. As it turned out, I had been doing everything back-tofront and upside down. I had been exercising without paying attention to my diet or any nutritional needs at all. I'd tried multiple brands of "skinny" pills, and had been riding a stationary bike for hours on end (with marginal results). I tried everything... Yep! I even starved myself with diets that gave temporary results. The stress of doing all of it with little to no results made me feel absolutely hopeless, worthless, and more than overly annoyed! I felt like completely giving up, many times. On so many occasions, in fact. I was lost and felt like I couldn't find my way out of it. I nearly gave up! Semi-depressed was my state of mind. It felt like everything sucked. I was very sad, mad, and exhausted. Now, I want to help as many people I can... because I've lost over 100 pounds!

I want to let you know, if you haven't already read my title, "How I Lost 100 Pounds! My Personal Weight Loss Strategies for Optimum Happiness," make sure you get your FREE copy today. Inside you'll learn exactly how I lost my weight, and the benefits of knowing the all the must-do nutrition, and other amazing secrets including myths, water weight, cellulite prevention and removal, the only exercise you really need, the ancient and easy technique to help slim you quickly, how to balance meals, and much, much more! I hope you love it. It's my very special gift to you!

I also want to let you know that I have been on my own, awesome health journey, utilizing amazing recipes like these (most of them I still use). And... I have managed to lose an enormous amount of weight, and, more importantly, keep it off, long term. So, I came to think; how can I share my knowledge with others? And what would be the best way to do so? Then, I realized that a book would be my best way... so here I am.

So, before we get into the amazing recipes, I want to show you some things that literally blew my mind! In Chapter 1, I will walk you through some of the sad health statistics in the US in our current time. Hopefully, you'll see just how important it is for you (and your family and loved ones) to take your health into your hands.

I especially want to share the information in Chapter 2 as well; and this relates to the benefits of using paleo as a real means to achieve weight loss. Ultimately, I want you to get a true benefit from reading this book, because I know how hard it is to lose weight, especially in the time we live in right now. So many "naughty" and "fast" foods, make it far too easy to go down the wrong path. I know because I did this for many years myself.

So, without further ado... let's get stuck in and start this journey together! I'll be here every single step of the way; cheering and motivating you, even during cooking times, energetically speaking, okay? I want you to know, that you really, truly, absolutely can do anything you set your mind too, and I know because I did it, and now here I am, hopefully helping you too! That's my aim. Let's go...

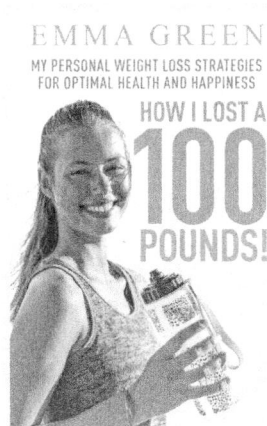

Btw check out "How i lost a 100 pounds" if you haven't already, its got loads of value and its completely FREE :)

FREE GIFTS!

Here are 3 bonus books I want to gift you for coming and reading this title! Sign up to my newsletter and you will receive:

Weight Loss Myths - 9 myths that you are mostly likely doing right now that are totally pointless and are a waste of time toward your weight loss goals.

How to Lose Weight Fast – A 10 day plan I personally put together to make that weight literally melt before your eyes (it worked for me!)

And... Weight Loss Secrets - Secrets the main stream media and health industry never talk about because (let's be honest) things that work don't make them money!

Click here to sign up! or for paperback versions grab it through the ebook completely FREE!

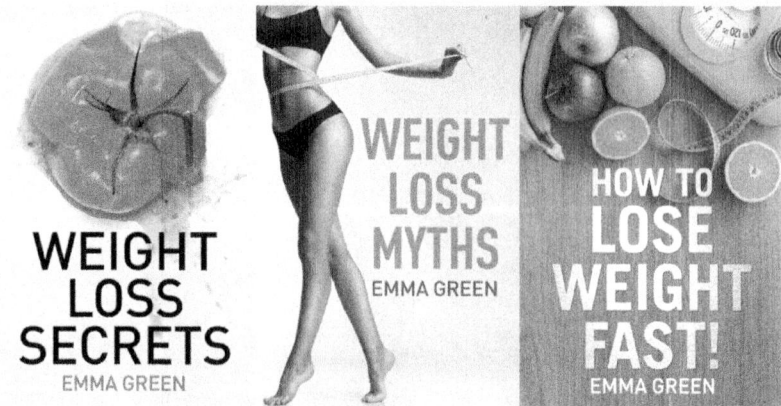

Chapter One

UNFORTUNATE HEALTH ISSUES FROM CONVENTIONAL US-BASED DIET

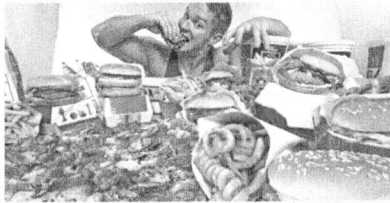

Let's take a look at some of the real statistics facing US adults and kids every day. Yes, the statistics are unfortunate, but through this knowledge I believe we can change the way we live. If we know how we can change the statistics, then we can truly do something about it and help future generations to change.

US Statistics:

More than 4 out of 10 cancer cases among adults in the United States can be prevented through diet and living factors. And almost half of all cancer-related deaths are associated with easily modifiable risk factors, a recent, American, Cancer Society study, indicates.

According to Farhad Islami, an MD with a PhD, and the Strategic Director of Cancer Surveillance Research for the American Cancer Society, in Atlanta, Georgia (and colleagues), "An estimated 42% of all cancer cases and nearly one-half of all cancer deaths in the United States in 2014 were attributable to evaluated risk factors, many of which could have been mitigated by effective preventive strategies. Our findings emphasize the continued need for widespread implementation of known preventive measures in the country to reduce the morbidity and premature mortality from cancers associated with potentially modifiable risk factors."

It's important to note that one of the biggest modifiable risk factors is, in fact, diet. And here we are trying to aid that factor.

Other breathtaking statistics show us that:

- Unhealthy diets contribute to 678,000 deaths per year in the US
- Obesity rates have doubled in the US for adults in the past 30 years
- Obesity rates have tripled in the US for children in the past 30 years
- Obesity rates have quadrupled in the US for adolescents in the past 30 years
- Recent reports project that half of all adults will be obese by the year 2030, and that's just in the US alone
- Poor eating habits and lack of physical activity are the top 2 reasons contributing to weight and obesity, globally

Okay, so now we have got that stuff out of the way, let's take a look at the benefits of using the paleo diet for weight loss and health. Then we can aid ourselves in being the best possible versions of ourselves, and feel good, too! Let's move onto Chapter 2 and see all the benefits of the paleo. You'll be pleasantly surprised by them! This is super-exciting!

Chapter Two

THE BENEFITS OF PALEO FOR WEIGHT LOSS

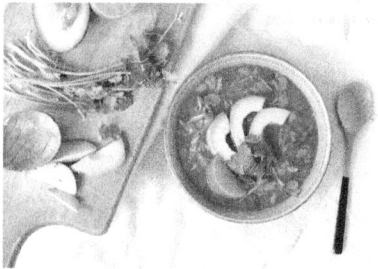

On a late, Saturday, summer afternoon, and when I usually had severe arthritic pain in my knees, I had a "lucky day." As usual, I had a rest in the afternoon and I watched TV, so I could put my feet up and relax. After an hour or so, I literally got up and walked around (ready to prepare a cup of tea) and I noticed that they felt much better; like to the point of having miniscule, nearly unnoticeable pain. I had been doing the paleo style for about two weeks and really thought that it was just "a lucky day" that I didn't feel the excruciating pain I normally did. Especially after a week of working hard.

The next day, I did the same on the Sunday. I sat down at about 3 pm and noticed that there was barely any pain at all. And, each day it diminished more, even during my work days. I was astonished at the difference that I felt, and I remember I became "nearly normal" again, in terms of symptomatic pain. When I thought about the "why" of it, I knew it must be from the nutritional change, because, in reality, everything else was pretty much the same, at that stage.

I investigated the healthful aspects of paleo, and its benefits online. I hadn't really done my homework on its health effects, apart from its benefit to weight loss. Because essentially, that was my main goal. One of the major aspects was its innate ability to crush inflammation, and another was that it helps with disease prevention. I was so excited, and I read and read, and found numerous studies on its benefits for health. To this day, I am so unbelievably grateful that my symptoms are (still) alleviated. Even my doctor was a little shocked, although I barely need to visit him much, anymore. No arguments here!

So yes, the paleo has been a definite go-to nutrition style for me, and I've now lost over 100 pounds as well. I did some other things too, but this nutrition was paramount in my overall efforts, especially in helping my arthritis and the inflammation associated with that. I know you'll love how easy it can be to do. Let's have a look together, now...

The paleo "mantra" is widely known as **no grains, no beans, no dairy, no sugar and no industrial seed oils**. And that is the easiest explanation I know. So, let's stick with that, shall we? Great!

So why the paleo?

It's important to know why we want to undertake it, especially if we want a health benefit or a weight loss one. So, let's look at the reasons why we should undertake it. The focus should be on vegetables, lean meats, fish chicken, and eggs. Fruit and nut consumption is kept to a minimum when on the paleo diet. Full fat products are allowed, and aren't calorie controlled.

The major benefits of the paleo diet include:

- Major weight loss over time
- Crushes inflammation in the body
- Helps disease prevention
- Can fully eliminate some diseases
- No calorie counting required
- Utilizes whole, non-processed foods
- Uses whole foods requiring less energy to digest
- It has similar benefits to the Mediterranean diet
- Scientifically proven to aid health
- Cardiovascular health improvements can be seen
- Effective in treating inflammatory bowel disease
- Effective in treating metabolic syndrome

Long-term diet risks:

- Compromised bone health through lack of calcium (which can be utilized elsewhere, in vegetable intake, as an example)
- High fish consumption (if toxins are present) can cause a build-up of toxins

So how does the paleo diet work?

The easiest way to understand the paleo (or paleolithic) diet is to realize that the predominant consumption of food is to utilize whole foods. Whole foods can be described as... foods that have not been processed or redefined (with additives or artificial substances and chemicals).

The paleo diet avoids dairy products, grains, sugar, legumes, processed oils, excess salt, alcohol, and coffee. The ideas behind the diet are founded by Walter Voegtlin and have been popularized by many dieticians and chefs very widely, and around the entire globe.

The paleo diet works to promote health. On a cellular level, it maneuvers food ingested, and in doing so, it begins improving the body's composition and its overall metabolic effects by way of substances taken in; noticeable in comparison to the high sugar/high salt diets profoundly demonstrated in the westernized culture. In fact, the paleo diet offers a wonderful alternative to the "dangerous" westernized diet, on the whole.

Chapter Three

PALEO BREAKFAST RECIPES

RECIPE#1: HEALTHY "NO-OAT" MEAL

Ingredients

- 1 small handful of walnuts
- 1 small handful of pecans
- 2 tablespoons of flax seed (ground)
- 1/2 – 1 teaspoon of cinnamon (ground)
- 1 pinch of nutmeg (ground)
- 1 pinch of ginger (ground)
- 1 tablespoon of almond butter
- 1 banana (mashed)
- 3 eggs
- 1/4 cup unsweetened of almond milk
- 2 teaspoons of pumpkin seeds
- 1 handful of fresh berries (choose seasonally)
- 1 tablespoon of organic honey

Instructions

- Add walnuts, pecans, and flax seed with spices to a processor. Blend until it's not totally ground into powder form.
- Whisk eggs and almond until consistency thickens to a loose custard.
- Thoroughly blend the mashed banana and almond butter and add it to the custard, mixing well as you go.
- Stir in the nutty mixture.
- Microwave or gently warm on the stovetop.
- Sprinkle pumpkin seeds and berries on top.

RECIPE#2: HASH WITH BRUSSELS

Ingredients

- 3 slices of bacon
- ½ a butternut squash
- ½ a red onion
- 1 clove of garlic
- 14 oz. of brussel sprouts
- 1 tablespoon of olive oil
- 4 eggs
- salt and pepper

Instructions

- Pan fry bacon in a skillet until crispy. Set aside on a separate plate.
- Chop butternut squash into cubes after peeling and de-seeding.
- Finely chop onion and brussel sprouts.
- Add to the pan the butternut squash and onion, and cook for 7 minutes, then stir in the brussel sprouts, mixing well.
- Sauté for a further 10 minutes, stirring as you go.
- Add the bacon to the pan, and mix well for 2 minutes, then add salt and pepper.

- Make 4 wells and crack an egg into each well, cover and sauté until eggs are set.

RECIPE#3: SANDWICH BONANZA

Ingredients

- 1 cup finely of ground unsweetened coconut
- 1 egg
- bacon
- mince patties
- bread

Instructions

- First you will need to make the coconut griddle cakes.
- Mix the fine coconut and the egg together.
- Cook on the stove like pancakes.
- Cook bacon and mince patties.
- Stack it in a sandwich.

Chapter Four

PALEO LUNCH RECIPES

Recipe#4: ITALIAN VEGETABLE LASAGNA

Ingredients

- 700g lean mince meat
- 1 onion, diced
- 2 garlic cloves (finely chopped)
- 5 tablespoons of rich tomato paste
- 30 oz. of diced tomato
- herbs – parsley, sage, mixed Italian herbs, thyme, basil, cumin ground, cinnamon
- 1 eggplant, sliced
- 1/4 butternut pumpkin, sliced
- 6 zucchinis, sliced
- 3 tablespoons of olive oil

Instructions

- Preheat oven to 180 degrees Celsius, fan-forced.
- Make sauce by frying onion and garlic in a pan until brown.
- Remove from pan, by placing in a bowl.
- Now add and cook the mince.

- When the mince is cooked, return the onion and garlic to the pan adding the herbs (to taste).
- Now add tomato paste and cook for 3 minutes.
- Add the diced tomatoes and leave to simmer on low heat for 30- 45 minutes.
- Layer eggplant slices along the bottom of an oven proof dish. Layer eggplant with 1/2 the mince sauce. Now layer with pumpkin slices, spreading the remaining mince sauce over the pumpkin; then layer zucchini slices on-top.
- Brush olive oil over zucchini slices.
- Bake for 30-40 minutes.

RECIPE#5: TASTY MOROCCAN SKEWERS

Ingredients

- 8 wooden skewers; soaked in cold water for 30 minutes
- 3 chicken breasts, diced

Marinade

- 1 garlic clove
- 2 teaspoons of honey
- 2 tablespoons of lemon juice
- 1 tablespoon of oil
- 1 teaspoon of cumin (ground)
- 1 teaspoon of salt
- 1/2 a teaspoon of cayenne pepper
- 1 teaspoon of turmeric (ground)
- 1/2 teaspoon of cinnamon (ground)
- pepper to taste

Instructions

- Dice chicken into cubes.
- Make marinade by combining ingredients in a small bowl,

mixing well. Put chicken in a large dish, pour marinade over the top and coat well. Cover and leave in the refrigerator overnight.
- Preheat oven to 180 degrees Celsius.
- Thread chicken onto skewers and place on an oven tray lined with baking paper.
- Slowly pour marinade over chicken.
- Bake for 35-40 minutes or until chicken is cooked properly.

RECIPE#6: CHILI AND GARLIC CHICKEN SKEWERS

Ingredients

- 8 wooden skewers; soaked in cold water for 30 minutes
- 3 chicken breasts, diced
- 2 tablespoons of olive oil
- 1 teaspoon of chopped red chilis
- 5 garlic cloves, finely chopped
- 6 tablespoons of lemon juice

Instructions

- Dice chicken into cubes.
- Make chili and garlic sauce by combining oil, chilis, garlic, and lemon juice in a small bowl, mixing well. Preheat oven to 180 degrees Celsius.
- Thread chicken onto skewers and place on an oven tray lined with baking paper.
- Slowly pour sauce over chicken, covering well.
- Bake for 35-40 minutes or until chicken is cooked properly.

RECIPE#7: YUMMY BOMBAY SKEWERS

Ingredients

- 8 wooden skewers; soaked in cold water for 30 minutes

- 3 chicken breasts, diced
- 4 tablespoons of oil
- 2 tablespoons of sweet paprika
- 1 tablespoon of coriander (ground)
- 1 tablespoon of cumin (ground)
- 1 tablespoon of turmeric (ground)
- 3 cloves of garlic, finely chopped

Instructions

- Preheat oven to 180 degrees Celsius.
- Make Bombay sauce by heating oil and all of the spices in a skillet for 2-3 minutes, or until fragrance is noticed.
- Thread chicken on skewers and place on an oven tray.
- Coat chicken well in sauce.
- Bake in oven for 30-40 minutes, or until chicken has cooked thoroughly.

RECIPE#8: SESAME SEED HONEY AND SOY CHICKEN

Ingredients

- 3 chicken breasts
- 1/2 a cup of honey
- 3 tablespoons of soy sauce
- 4 tablespoons of sesame seeds

Instructions

- Preheat oven to 180 degrees Celsius, fan-forced.
- Mix the honey and soy sauce, add chicken and coat thickly.
- Place chicken and sauce on a baking tray, lined with baking paper.
- Place in oven and cook for 12 minutes.
- Remove from oven; add sesame seeds (as much or as little as you like).

- Return to oven and cook for a further 10 minutes or until chicken has cooked thoroughly.

RECIPE#9: DELICIOUS CHICKEN SATAYS

Ingredients

- 3 chicken breasts
- 1 tablespoon of coriander (ground)
- 1 tablespoon of turmeric (ground)
- 1 onion, chopped
- 3 cloves of garlic, finely chopped
- 4 tablespoons of olive oil
- Garam masala (to taste)
- A squeeze of lemon (to taste)

Instructions

- Place olive oil, lemon juice, onion, garlic cloves, coriander, turmeric, and garam masala into processor. Blend together on high until a very smooth texture is formed.
- Thread chicken onto wooden skewers and put in a bowl, pour marinade over chicken, turning until coated well. Cover and place in the refrigerator for 1-2 hours to permeate flavors.
- Preheat oven to 180 degrees Celsius, fan-forced.
- Put chicken skewers on an oven proof tray lined with baking paper, then lovingly brush with marinade.
- Bake in oven for 20-30 minutes until chicken has cooked thoroughly.

RECIPE#10: CHICKEN ALFREDO WITH CASHEWS

Ingredients

- 1 lb. chicken breast

- 1 x 12 oz. packet of kelp noodles
- 5 cloves of garlic, chopped
- 3 teaspoons of olive oil
- 2 teaspoons of tarragon
- 1 cup of cashews
- 1/2 teaspoon of onion powder
- 1/4 teaspoon of garlic powder
- 1/4 teaspoon of mustard powder
- 1/4 teaspoon of sea salt
- 1/4 teaspoon of pepper
- 1/8 teaspoon of paprika (ground)

Instructions

- Add the olive oil to a large skillet. Lightly cook the garlic over medium heat for approximately 4 minutes.
- Chop the chicken into 2-inch cubes, then add to the skillet and cook until brown.
- Rinse and chop noodles. Add them to the skillet along with the tarragon. Now cover and cook for 30 minutes on low heat.
- Pour the liquid from the skillet carefully into a small container for use in the sauce.
- Add the cashews, the onion powder, the garlic powder, the mustard powder, the salt, the pepper, and the ground paprika to be blended into a powder.
- Add the (reserved) pan juices very slowly, making a thickened sauce.
- Add the sauce to the skillet, then mix well. Cover and continue to cook for 12 minutes on a low to medium heat.

RECIPE#11: DELIGHTFUL MOROCCAN CASSEROLE

Ingredients

- 1 head of cauliflower

- 2-3 lb. of chicken
- 2 tablespoons of butter
- 1 onion, finely chopped
- 2 tablespoons ginger root, finely chopped
- 2 garlic cloves, finely chopped
- 3 carrots, peeled and sliced
- 2 teaspoons of cumin
- 1 teaspoon of paprika
- 1 teaspoon of coriander
- 1/2 teaspoon of turmeric
- 1/2 teaspoon of cinnamon
- 1/4 tsp of cayenne
- 1 bell pepper, cut into thin strips
- 1 x 28 oz. can of diced tomatoes (with juice)
- 1/2 cup of minced parsley or cilantro
- 2 teaspoons of salt
- 1 lemon

Instructions

- Preheat oven to 180 degrees Celsius.
- Chop the head of the cauliflower into smaller pieces. Place through a food processor using the grating blade.
- Spread cauliflower out in a rectangular baking pan.
- Add salt and pepper to the chicken. Melt down 1 tablespoon of butter in a deep pan over a medium heat. Add the chicken, browning it.
- Remove the chicken and set aside. Turn heat down to medium and place in the onion, ginger, garlic and carrots.
- Cook until the onions are light brown. Add remaining tablespoon of butter spices. Mix together well.
- Add bell pepper, the can of tomatoes, minced parsley (or cilantro) and salt.
- Return the chicken and simmer for 5 minutes.
- Pour the mixture over the cauliflower and mix well, so the

cauliflower is completely covered by the sauce. Slice a lemon and lay it evenly on top of the casserole.
- Cover the pan with tin foil and bake for 40 minutes.
- Remove the tinfoil and cook for 20 minutes more.

RECIPE#12: BEEF AND MUSHROOM GOULASH

Ingredients

- 1 lb. of diced beef
- 2 tablespoons of olive oil
- 1 onion, diced
- 8 oz. button mushrooms, sliced
- 3 tablespoons of paprika (ground)
- a 1 and a 1/2 (14.5 oz.) can of diced tomatoes
- parsley (as garnish)
- salt
- pepper

Instructions

- In a medium pan, fry 1/2 the beef in 1 tablespoon of oil for 5 minutes, or until brown.
- Move beef to a plate and repeat process with remaining beef.
- Place remaining oil into the pan.
- Add onion and mushrooms, then cook while stirring for 4 minutes or until tender.
- Add the paprika and mix well to coat the mushrooms and onions.
- Add in the tomatoes and beef.
- Cover them and leave to simmer for 15 minutes.
- Add salt and pepper before serving with the chopped parsley, used as a garnish.

RECIPE #13: MASTERFUL MEATBALLS:

Meatballs

- 2 tablespoons of olive oil
- 1 onion, diced
- 1 lb. of lean mince meat
- 2 garlic cloves, finely diced
- 1 apple, grated
- 1/4 of a cup of raisins
- 8 black olives, chopped
- 3 tablespoons of slivered almonds
- 1 egg
- a dash of cinnamon
- a dash of cloves
- 1 teaspoon of chili powder
- salt and pepper (to taste)

Ingredients
Sauce

- 1 x 28 oz. can of diced tomatoes
- a dash of cinnamon
- a dash of cloves
- a dash of paprika

Instructions

- Preheat oven to 180 degrees Celsius, fan forced.
- Heat the oil and fry onion until brown.
- Add to the beef; the garlic, apple, raisins, olives, almonds, egg, cinnamon, cloves, chili powder, salt, and pepper. Combine ingredients well.
- Form the mixture into 14 balls.
- Now bake in the preheated oven for 15-20 minutes, or until cooked and brown.

- While the meatballs are baking, place the tomatoes, cinnamon, cloves, and paprika into a pan to simmer.
- Add meatballs to pan for a further 15-20 minutes.

RECIPE#14: SCRUMPTIOUS MEAT LOAF

Ingredients

- 1 zucchini
- 3 small carrots
- 1/2 a cup of peas
- 1 small onion, finely diced
- 1 lb. of mince
- 1 egg
- 1 teaspoon of mixed Italian herbs
- 1/2 a teaspoon of salt

Instructions

- Preheat oven to 180 degrees Celsius, fan -forced.
- Grate carrots and zucchini, and squeeze to remove as much liquid as possible.
- Put carrots and zucchini into a large mixing bowl along with peas, onion, mince, egg, herbs, and salt. Mix together well.
- Using a muffin-type tray, line each individual hole with baking paper. Tightly pack the mince mixture into each space.
- Bake in the oven for 35 -40 minutes, or until cooked well-through.

RECIPE#15: LAMB AND MUSHROOM SKEWERS

Ingredients

- 6 wooden skewers; soaked in cold water for 30 minutes
- 1 lb. of diced lamb

- 20 button mushrooms
- 4 tablespoons of olive oil
- 2 teaspoons of honey
- 1/2 teaspoon of rosemary leaves, finely chopped
- 1 garlic clove, finely chopped
- salt and pepper (to taste)

Instructions

- Preheat oven to 180 degrees Celsius, fan-forced.
- Place olive oil, honey, rosemary, garlic, and the salt and pepper in a bowl and mix together well.
- Thread lamb onto skewers with mushrooms, changing as you go.
- Place on oven tray (lined)
- Coat with olive oil and the honey sauce.
- Place in oven for approximately 40 minutes, or until lamb has cooked thoroughly through.

RECIPE #16: SPICY MEATBALLS WITH FLAMING CHILI SAUCE

Ingredients

- 1/4 lb. of lean, mince
- 3 tablespoons of cooked brown rice
- 1/4 of a teaspoon of dried parsley
- 1/4 of a teaspoon of Italian seasoning
- 1/4 of a teaspoon of fennel seeds
- 1/8 of a teaspoon of garlic powder
- 1/8 of a teaspoon of red-pepper flakes
- 1/8 of a teaspoon of dried minced onion
- a pinch of salt
- a pinch of black pepper
- 2 and a 1/2 tablespoons of chili sauce
- 1/8 of a teaspoon of hot-pepper sauce, or more

Instructions

- Preheat the oven to 180 degrees Celsius.
- In a large bowl, combine the beef and rice, then the parsley, Italian seasoning, fennel, garlic powder, red-pepper flakes, onion, salt, and pepper.
- Mix well.
- Form medium-sized balls.
- Place the meatballs in a single layer on a small, nonstick baking sheet.
- Bake for 8 minutes.
- Transfer to a medium bowl and set aside.
- In a separate bowl, combine the chili sauce with the hot-pepper sauce.
- Pour the sauce over the meatballs.

RECIPE#17: DUMPLINGS OF LAMB AND BACON

Meatballs

- 8 pieces of bacon meat, finely diced
- 1 onion, finely chopped
- 1 tablespoon of oil
- 2 teaspoons of sage, finely chopped
- 1 teaspoon of paprika (ground)
- salt and pepper
- 1 lb. of minced lamb
- 1 egg
- sauce
- 2 cans of diced tomatoes
- 4 cups of freshly diced tomatoes
- 1 teaspoon of basil, finely chopped
- salt and pepper

Instructions

- Preheat oven to 180 degrees Celsius, fan-forced.
- Fry onion and bacon for 6 minutes, or until onion becomes tender.
- Add the paprika, sage, salt and pepper, and cook for a further 3 minutes, then remove from heat.
- In another bowl, add the (now-cooled) bacon mixture and egg to the minced lamb, mixing well.
- Roll lamb mixture into 14 balls and place on baking tray, lined.
- Bake in the oven for 35-40 minutes, or until cooked.
- For the sauce; place diced tomatoes, basil, salt and pepper in a medium sized pan and simmer for 3 minutes.
- Add the cooked meatballs and simmer for a further 8-10 minutes.

RECIPE#18: MOROCCAN LAMB

Ingredients

- 1 lb. of diced lamb
- 1 tablespoon of oil
- 3 cups of chicken stock
- 1 tablespoon of cinnamon (ground)
- 4 cups of diced pumpkin
- 1 onion, sliced
- 8 yellow, button squash, cut into halves
- 1 lemon, juiced
- 1 tablespoon of honey
- 2/3 of a cup of pitted prunes
- a pinch of salt and pepper

Instructions

- Heat oil and fry diced lamb until cooked.
- Add the chicken stock and then the cinnamon.
- Simmer for 1 hour.

- Add pumpkin, squash, onion, lemon juice and honey. Then cover and simmer for another 25 minutes. Make sure vegetables are cooked.
- Add in the prunes, salt and pepper to taste, and cook for 6 minutes.

RECIPE#19: EGGPLANT EXTRAVAGANZA

Ingredients

- 1/3 of a lb. of lean mince
- 1/2 a cup of diced onion
- 4 garlic cloves (finely chopped)
- 1 tablespoon of tomato paste
- 14.5 oz. diced tomato
- herbs – sage, mixed Italian herbs, thyme, basil, cumin, ground cinnamon
- 1 eggplant (cut in half)
- 1 cup of lettuce

Instructions

- Add eggplant halves into a baking tray and bake in a preheated 180-degree Celsius oven. Do this for 20 minutes, or until soft.
- Now fry the onion and garlic in a pan until brown.
- Remove from the pan and cook the mince, stirring well for a better consistency.
- When the mince is cooked, return the onion and garlic to the pan.
- Add herbs (to taste).
- Add in tomato paste and cook for 3 minutes. Add in the diced tomatoes and leave to simmer for 25 minutes.
- When the eggplant is done, use a fork to scrape the inside of the eggplant until it's soft and squishy, Place the mince on top of the eggplant half and just serve with lettuce.

RECIPE#20: AMAZING ORANGE CHICKEN

Sauce

- 1 carton of 100% orange juice
- 1 tablespoon of Szechuan sauce
- 2 tablespoons of organic honey
- 1 tablespoon of coconut flour

Instructions

- Whisk all of the ingredients together in a saucepan and allow it to come to a boil. Lower temperature and simmer slowly.
- Now whisking occasionally, for 20 minutes, or until reduced by half original size.

Ingredients
Chicken

- 3 chicken breasts, thawed
- 1/4 of a cup of almond flour
- 1/4 of a cup of flaxseed meal
- 1/2 teaspoon of chili powder
- 1/2 teaspoon of garlic
- 1/2 teaspoon of oregano
- 1/4 teaspoon of sea salt

Instructions

- Preheat oven to 200 degrees Celsius.
- Pat chicken dry and cut into bite-sized pieces.
- Combine the last 6 ingredients together in a large sized zip-lock bag.
- Place chicken pieces into a bag and toss to coat.
- Remove and place on foil-lined baking sheet.

- Bake for 15-20 minutes.
- Now drizzle with orange sauce to your liking.

RECIPE#21: GREEN CHILI CHICKEN

Ingredients

- 2 lb. boneless skinless chicken breasts, cut into chunks
- 1 tablespoon of coconut flour
- 1 1/2 tablespoons of coconut oil
- 1/2 an onion
- 2 cloves of garlic, minced
- 1 tablespoon of cumin (ground)
- 1 1/2 teaspoons of dried oregano
- 1 teaspoon of chipotle chili powder
- 1/2 lb. of spinach leaves
- 1 cup of chicken stock (made)
- 1 sweet potato, roasted and mashed
- 6 tomatillos, cut into chunks
- 1 x 14 oz. can of diced green chilis

Instructions

- Place chunked chicken breasts into a bowl with 1 tablespoon of coconut flour and salt and pepper to taste.
- Mix until well-distributed.
- Heat the oil in a Dutch oven over medium heat.
- Add the onion and sauté until onion is soft.
- Add garlic and sauté for a further 30 seconds.
- Turn heat to medium and add chicken and spices. Cook until chicken has no more pink showing.
- Add the tomatillos and the green chilis, then add the stock and spinach, bringing to a simmer.
- Reduce heat and allow to simmer for about 30 minutes, stirring occasionally.

- Add mashed sweet potato and mix well. Return to a simmer and serve.
- Roast sweet potatoes, for 30-45 minutes directly on the oven rack until easily pierced with a fork. Serve with chicken.
- 4 oz. of light cream cheese, room temperature1 (15 oz.) can of diced tomatoes, well drained
- 1/2 a cup of frozen corn kernels
- 1 (4 oz.) can of green chilies, roasted and chopped
- salt and pepper
- 4 organic, boneless, skinless chicken breasts
- olive oil
- Tajin seasoning (a blend of dehydrated lime, ground chilis peppers and salt to taste)

Instructions

- Preheat oven to 220 degrees Celsius.
- In a bowl, use an electric mixer on low speed, to combine the cream cheese, drained tomatoes, corn and the chilis.
- Slice through the thick part of each chicken breast so that it opens (like a book).
- Doubly-wrap the chicken with plastic wrap, and then bash it out with a meat mallet until it's 1/2 to 1/4 inches in thickness.
- Season one side of each chicken breast with salt and pepper, then flip it over and spread with 1/4 of the cream.
- For cheese filling: roll each chicken breast up and place it seam-side down in a baking dish. Rub over some olive oil.
- Cover the top of the chicken then season with Tajin, and then add the salt and pepper.
- Cover and bake for 40 minutes.
- Remove the cover and bake for another 12 minutes.
- Thinly slice before you serve.

RECIPE#23: FRIED CHICKEN WITH HERBS

Ingredients

- 2 eggs
- 2 tablespoons of fruit-only apricot preserves
- 2 tablespoons of Dijon mustard
- 1/2 a teaspoon of garlic powder
- 1/2 a teaspoon of red pepper flakes
- 1/2 a cup of almond flour
- 1/2 a cup of almond meal
- 1/2 a cup of coconut flour
- 1/2 a teaspoon of black pepper
- 1/2 a teaspoon of dried thyme
- 1/2 a teaspoon of sweet paprika
- 1/2 a teaspoon of salt
- 2 lbs. of boneless, skinless, chicken tenders

Instructions

- Preheat oven to 220 degrees Celsius.
- Lightly grease a 13″x 9″ baking pan with coconut oil.
- In a bowl, whisk the eggs, the apricot preserves, the mustard, the garlic powder, and the red pepper flakes.
- In another bowl, combine the almond flour, almond meal, coconut flour, pepper, thyme, paprika and then the salt.
- Dip each chicken piece into the egg mixture, then put through the flour mixture. Place in the pre-prepared pan.
- Bake for 40 minutes.
- Change oven to high-broil for 2 minutes and turn each chicken piece, then broil the other side for 2 minutes.

RECIPE#24: SQUASH-CASSEROLE SPAGHETTI

Ingredients

- 1 spaghetti squash
- 1 tablespoon of olive oil
- 4 cloves of garlic
- 1 sweet onion, chopped
- 2 zucchinis, chopped
- 2 tomatoes, chopped
- 1/3 of a cup of basil leaves, chopped
- 2 teaspoons of dried oregano
- 1 jar of spaghetti sauce
- a large handful of shredded soy cheese

Instructions

- Preheat oven to 220 degrees Celsius.
- Cut spaghetti squash in half and scoop out the seeds.
- Wash the squash with water, then microwave each half individually for 5 1/2 minutes.
- Heat olive oil in a large pan over medium heat. Add garlic. After a few minutes add onion.
- After a few more minutes add zucchini. Finally add tomatoes, basil and oregano, and cook for another 6 minutes.
- Scoop out the spaghetti squash and place in a large mixing bowl. Add the veggies from the pan. Pour the entire jar of spaghetti squash into the bowl and mix well.
- Place the squash mixture into a large baking dish, and top with cheese and bake for 25 minutes.

RECIPE#25: YUMMY STUFFED CHICKEN WITH POTATO

Ingredients

- 4 oz. of light cream cheese, room temperature
- 1 (15 oz.) can diced tomatoes, drained
- 1/2 cup frozen corn kernels
- 1 (4 oz.) can of green chilies, roasted and chopped

- salt and pepper
- 4, boneless, skinless, chicken breasts
- olive oil
- Tajin seasoning (a blend of dehydrated lime, ground chili peppers and salt to taste)
- 4 potatoes (baked)
- 1 tub of sour cream
- 1 tablespoon of chives, chopped

Instructions

- Preheat oven to 220 degrees Celsius.
- In a bowl, use an electric mixer on low speed, to combine the cream cheese, drained tomatoes, corn and the chilis.
- Slice through the thick part of each chicken breast so that it opens (like a book).
- Doubly-wrap the chicken with plastic wrap, and then bash it out with a meat mallet until it's 1/2 to 1/4 inches in thickness.
- Season one side of each chicken breast with salt and pepper, then flip it over and spread with 1/4 of the cream.
- For cheese filling: roll each chicken breast up and place it seam-side down in a baking dish. Rub over some olive oil.
- Cover the top of the chicken then season with Tajin, and then add the salt and pepper.
- Cover and bake for 40 minutes.
- Remove the cover and bake for another 12 minutes.
- Thinly slice before you serve.
- Bake potatoes for 40 minutes and add sour cream to taste. Add chives.

RECIPE#26: STUFFED TURKEY WITH PEPPERS

Ingredients

- 5 bell peppers

- 1 tablespoon of olive oil
- 2 cloves of garlic
- 2 tablespoons of fresh basil, minced
- 1 onion, minced
- 1 tablespoon of fresh rosemary, dried
- 1 teaspoon of dried parsley
- a dash of salt and pepper
- 20 oz. of organic (ground) turkey
- 1 tomato, chopped
- 3/4 of a cup of spaghetti sauce
- 1/2 a cup of shredded mozzarella cheese

Instructions

- Bring a large pot of water to boil, then add a pinch of salt. Cut tops off the bell peppers and remove the seeds.
- Place in boiling water, using a spoon to keep them submerged until softened. Drain and set aside.
- Preheat the oven to 180 degrees Celsius. Prepare a baking pan.
- In a large pan, heat the oil on medium. Add the garlic, basil, onion, rosemary, parsley, and then the salt and pepper.
- Cook for 6 minutes, or until the onions begin to soften.
- Add the ground turkey and continue to heat.
- Add the tomato and cook for another 3 minutes.
- Remove from the heat.
- Now add the spaghetti sauce into the turkey mixture and mix well.
- Add the cheese and mix in.
- Stuff each bell pepper with the turkey mixture and place on the baking sheet.
- Cook for 20 minutes, or until the bell peppers become soft.

RECIPE#27: SLOW COOKER CABBAGE SOUP

Ingredients

- 1 lb. ground beef
- 4 cups of red and green cabbage, chopped
- 3 carrots, diced
- 1 onion, diced
- 2 cups of fresh tomatoes, chopped
- 4 garlic cloves, minced
- 2 cups of tomato sauce
- 5 cups of beef or chicken stock
- 1 teaspoon of paprika
- 1 teaspoon of dried oregano
- 1/2 a teaspoon of dried basil
- cooking fat (lard or butter)
- salt and black pepper (ground)

Instructions

- Melt the cooking fat in a pan on medium to high heat.
- Add the garlic and onion and cook for 3 minutes, then add the beef.
- Cook the beef until brown; season beef with paprika, then add salt and pepper (to taste).
- Place the beef in a slow cooker, and add all the remaining ingredients in.
- Adjust the seasoning to taste and mix everything well.
- Cover and cook on low for 6 to 7 hours, (or on high for 5 hours).

Chapter Five

PALEO DINNER RECIPES

Recipe#28: PORK WITH HONEY AND APPLE

Ingredients

- 50g of olive oil
- 1/4 cup honey
- 8 x 1/2 lb. pork fillet (pieces)
- 4 pink lady apples, sliced horizontally into thin slices
- a pinch of chopped sage
- 3 bunches of spinach
- 4 tablespoons of pine nuts
- a squeeze of lemon juice
- salt and pepper

Instructions

- Preheat oven to 180 degrees Celsius.
- Combine olive oil and honey over a low heat until honey has melted. Glaze the pork in the honey, dipping well, cooking both sides for around 3 minutes.
- Now, on a baking tray, lay out 8 groups of 4 apple slices

(approx.) and brush with honey mixture, then add the sage and the pork.
- Top with 2 or 3 more apple slices and another coat of honey as required.
- Bake for 20 minutes, or until the apples have caramelized.
- Separately, (in a fry pan on low heat) place in pine nuts and stir until brown.
- Steam the spinach until cooked and mix in a squeeze of lemon juice to taste.
- To serve, place pine nuts on top of spinach as a complementing side dish to the pork main.

RECIPE#29: PIZZA PALEO

Ingredients

- 3 teaspoons of olive oil, divided
- 1 cup of almonds (ground) or other nut choice (to taste)
- 3 tablespoons of cashews (ground) butter
- 1/3 of a cup of egg white
- 1/2 cup of onion, chopped
- 2 cloves of minced garlic
- 1 chopped red pepper
- 1/2 cup of halved grape tomatoes
- 1 large Italian sausage, cut into 1/2" slices
- 1/2 cup of marinara sauce
- 1/2 teaspoon of oregano

Instructions

- Mix ground nuts, cashew butter, and egg whites in a large bowl.
- Grease a pizza sheet with 2 teaspoons of the olive oil, then spread the dough mixture over it, making a thick crust.
- Preheat the oven to 180 degrees Celsius.

- In a pan, add the remaining olive oil and the slices of sausage.
- Cook until brown, then remove the sausage once cooked.
- Add the garlic, the onions, and red pepper to the pan. Sauté the vegetables lightly, but not so they are too soft.
- Cover the dough with the marinara sauce, then add the meat and vegetables, excluding the tomatoes.
- Add the oregano, then bake for 25 minutes.
- Remove from oven, adding the halved tomatoes, and serve.

RECIPE#30: HEARTY SHEPHERD'S PIE

Ingredients

- 1 head of cauliflower
- 2 tablespoons of butter
- 1-3 tablespoons of cream
- salt pepper
- 4 tablespoons of olive oil
- 1 onion, chopped
- 1 cup of frozen peas and carrots, thawed
- 3/4 of a cup of frozen green beans, thawed
- 1 lb. of beef
- 1 tablespoon of coconut flour or almond flour
- 3/4 of a cup of beef stock
- 1 tablespoon of chopped fresh thyme
- 1 tablespoon chopped fresh rosemary
- 2 tablespoons of butter

Instructions

- Preheat oven to 200 degrees Celsius.
- Break the cauliflower into chunky pieces and steam until tender.
- Using a food processor, add it in, with 2 tablespoons of

butter and blending until smooth. Add salt and pepper to taste.

- Add cream a tablespoon at a time, do this until smooth and thick. Set aside.
- Heat oil in a pan over medium to low heat. Add onion, cooking until soft.
- Add beef and cook for about 5 minutes, stirring to break up the meat so it browns.
- Add in peas, carrots and green beans and cook for 6 minutes.
- Stir in the coconut flour.
- Add stock and herbs and reduce and simmer, stirring occasionally, for 5 minutes.
- Add salt and pepper.
- Remove from pan and put into a large pie pan (glass or other). Spread the cauliflower over the top as a covering.
- Add 2 tablespoons of butter and cut into small pieces on top of the cauliflower.
- Bake for 35 minutes.

RECIPE#31: BEAUTIFUL BURGUNDY BEEF

Ingredients

- 1/4 lb. of bacon
- 4 tablespoons of butter
- 2 1/2 to 3 lbs. of beef cut into 2-inch cubes.
- 1 1/2 teaspoons of salt
- 1/4 of a teaspoon of pepper
- 2 tablespoons of almond flour
- 2 carrots, sliced
- 1 onion, sliced
- 1 tablespoon of tomato paste
- 3 cloves of garlic, finely chopped
- 1 tablespoon of fresh thyme
- 1 tablespoon of fresh parsley, finely chopped

- 3 cups of red wine
- 2 and a 1/2 cups of beef stock
- 1 lb. of white or brown mushrooms

Instructions

- Preheat oven to 200 degrees Celsius.
- Cut bacon into short strips.
- Sauté the bacon in 1 tablespoon of butter.
- Add beef to the bacon in 3-4 batches. Brown each batch then remove from pan.
- Set bacon and meat aside in the baking dish you will use in the oven.
- Add salt, pepper and almond flour evenly over the meat.
- Bake meat in the oven without a cover for 10 minutes.
- Remove from the oven and turn the heat down to 160 degrees Celsius.
- In a separate saucepan, add 1 tablespoon of butter to the remaining fat from the bacon and meat, and then sauté the carrots and onion until soft, for about 10 minutes.
- Add the tomato paste, garlic, thyme, and parsley.
- Stir in the wine and the stock and bring to a gentle boil. Let simmer for 5 minutes, then pour over the meat in the casserole pan.
- Cover the dish and cook for about 2 and a half hours. The liquid should be gently bubbling the whole time.
- Slice the mushrooms and sauté in the remaining tablespoons of butter.
- When the meat is done, remove from the oven.
- Put a bowl under a colander and pour the meat and liquid into the colander to drain out liquid. Be careful of the heat.
- Bring the liquid to a slow boil and simmer for 10 minutes. Pour over meat and mushrooms.
- Garnish with parsley.

RECIPE#32: SPINACH-PLUS PINWHEELS

Ingredients

- 1 cup of fresh spinach leaves
- 1/2 (14-ounce) can of artichokes, chopped
- 1 tablespoon of grated parmesan cheese
- 1 clove of garlic, minced
- 1 tablespoon of fresh parsley (chopped)
- 2 tablespoons of Italian-style bread crumbs
- 1 tablespoon of olive oil
- 1 1/2 lbs. of lean, flank steak

Instructions

- Combine spinach with breadcrumbs in a bowl.
- Stir in 1 teaspoon of oil.
- Pound steak to 1/2 an inch to allow for movement when rolling.
- Place the steak in a baking dish.
- Scatter spinach mixture (with all other ingredients well mixed) evenly over the steak. Starting with the longest edge, roll up steak, and tie tightly with some string to secure.
- Heat the remainder of the oil in a large pan over medium to high heat.
- Brown steak for 5 minutes, both sides.
- Place steak on a baking sheet and bake at 220 degrees Celsius for 15 minutes, or until done to taste.
- Let steak rest for 4 minutes.
- Remove string and slice evenly.

RECIPE#33: SWEET POTATO AND TUNA PATTIES

Ingredients

- 2 cups of diced sweet potato, peeled

- 180g can of tuna in brine, drained
- 1/4 of a cup of almond meal
- 2 eggs
- 1 tablespoon of olive oil
- salt and pepper

Instructions

- Place diced sweet potato in a pan with water on medium heat and boil for 15 minutes.
- Remove sweet potato and place in a mixing bowl along with tuna, almond meal, eggs, olive oil, and the salt and pepper.
- Combine well.
- Shape mixture into patties and place on a preheated grill on medium heat.
- Cook for 5-7 minutes.

RECIPE#34: KING SALMON WITH CHANTERELLE MUSHROOMS

Ingredients

- 4 pieces of king salmon steaks (with center cut, 10 ounces each)
- 1/2 a pound of chanterelle mushrooms, sliced
- 4 ounces of olive oil, divided
- 6 ounces of white wine
- 16 ounces of chicken stock
- 1/2 a tablespoon of fresh thyme, chopped
- 2 tablespoons of minced shallots
- 1 tablespoon of minced garlic
- 3 tablespoons of whole butter, divided
- 1 tablespoon of fresh lemon juice
- salt and black pepper
- lemon (wedges) and parsley

Instructions

- Preheat grill to medium heat.
- Brush salmon filets with 1 ounce of olive oil and season well with salt and black pepper.
- Grill fish to taste.
- Separately, preheat a large heavy pan over high heat and add the remaining 3 ounces of olive oil. When oil is hot, add the mushrooms and add salt and pepper.
- Remove pan from heat after 2 minutes.
- Turn the mushrooms. When slightly brown on the second side, empty the mushrooms into a strainer with a pan underneath to catch oil.
- Return the pan to the heat and add 1 tablespoon of butter to the pan. Add shallots and garlic.
- Add thyme. Remove from heat and use white wine.
- Return to heat and reduce liquid by half.
- When reduced, add stock and reduce to saucy consistency.
- Return mushrooms to pan and add the remainder of the whole butter. Swirl the pan until butter is completely melted.
- Remove the salmon from the grill and place on a large serving platter.
- Top the salmon filets with the mushroom mixture, and garnish with lemons and parsley as required.

RECIPE#35: ROASTED PUMPKIN SOUP

Ingredients

- 4 lb. of diced pumpkin
- 1 garlic bulb, un-peeled
- 2 tablespoons of olive oil
- 1 large onion, diced
- 3 tablespoons of cumin (ground)
- 3 cups of vegetable stock
- 1 good bunch of fresh basil, chopped
- salt and pepper

Instructions

- Preheat oven to 180 degrees Celsius, fan-forced.
- Place garlic on an oven tray and drizzle the olive oil.
- Place diced pumpkin on the same tray around the garlic.
- Use oven and bake for 45 minutes, or until vegetables are tender.
- Remove from oven and cool slightly before peeling garlic.
- Fry onion in a large pan with the remaining oil for 3 minutes.
- Add cumin and stir.
- Add stock, pumpkin and garlic cloves and simmer for 12 to 14 minutes. Stir every 2 minutes.
- Remove from heat and add salt and pepper.

RECIPE#36: HOMEMADE LEEK AND GARLIC SOUP

Ingredients

- 4 bulbs of garlic
- 4 leeks (white part only)
- 1 onion, chopped
- 4 cups of chicken or vegetable stock
- ¾ of a cup of coconut milk
- olive oil

Instructions

- Preheat oven to 180 degrees Celsius, fan-forced.
- Place garlic bulb top down on an oven tray, and drizzle olive oil.
- Place in the oven for 35-40minutes.
- Remove from oven and leave to cool.
- Fry up the onion and leek in a pan with the oil on a medium heat for 12 minutes.
- Add stock and simmer for a further 12 minutes.

- Remove from heat and add the garlic and the coconut milk to the pan.
- Use an electric blender to blend the soup into a smooth texture.
- Heat before serving.

RECIPE#37: CRISPY CAJUN FRIES WITH SALAD

Ingredients

- 1 butternut squash
- 1/2 a teaspoon of olive oil
- 1 teaspoon of paprika
- 1/8 of a teaspoon cayenne
- 1/8 of a teaspoon of garlic powder
- 1/8 of a teaspoon of onion powder
- 1/8 of a teaspoon of salt

Ingredients
Salad

- 1/2 a lettuce
- 1 cucumber
- a handful of alfalfa
- 1 red onion
- 2 carrots
- balsamic vinegar

Instructions

- Preheat the oven to 220 degrees Celsius.
- Carefully cut both ends off the squash.
- Peel the rind from the squash and discard the rind.
- Cut the squash in halves, lengthwise. Now, scrape out the seeds and discard their 8 ounces (approx. 2 cups). You can

refrigerate the remainder of the squash for another recipe if you wish.
- Place the squash sticks in a mixing bowl.
- Add the oil, paprika, cayenne, garlic powder, onion powder, and salt. Toss and coat.
- Transfer them to a baking sheet so the sticks are in a single layer.
- Bake, and turn the squash about every 4 minutes, for 24 minutes, or until crisp.
- Chop up salad ingredients and toss, add balsamic vinegar to taste.

RECIPE#38: ROASTED BUTTERNUT AND SQUASH WITH PAPRIKA

Ingredients

- 1 large butternut squash
- 1 teaspoon of sweet paprika
- 1 teaspoon of garlic powder
- 1 teaspoon of onion salt
- 1 teaspoon of black pepper (ground)
- 2 teaspoons of balsamic vinegar
- 3 tablespoons of olive oil

Instructions

- Preheat oven to 200 degrees Celsius.
- Cut ends off butternut squash, peel, and slice in lengths.
- Remove seeds and chop into 1-inch cubes.
- In a ceramic bowl, combine spices, and the oil and vinegar into a paste.
- Add squash and toss until coated.
- Arrange the cubes of squash in one layer in a roasting pan.
- Roast for 25 minutes, toss, and cook for an additional 20 minutes or until the squash is tender.

RECIPE#39: PORTOBELLO ROAST BEEF

Ingredients

- 2 1/2 lbs. beef rib roast
- 2 cups beef stock
- 2 Portobello mushrooms, sliced
- 1/4 of a cup of balsamic vinegar
- 2 tablespoons of onion flakes
- 1 tablespoons of garlic flakes
- 1 tablespoon of dried oregano
- sea salt and black pepper (ground)

Instructions

- Preheat your oven to 220 degrees Celsius.
- In a medium-sized bowl, combine the garlic, onion, oregano, and salt and pepper; this is the seasoning.
- Rub the seasoning all over the roast.
- Place the roast on a rack in the oven in a roasting pan.
- Roast uncovered, for about 2 hours.
- Take the roast out of the pan, but don't rinse out the pan. Set the roast aside to rest for about 12 minutes.
- While the meat rests, heat the roasting pan on the stovetop over low to medium heat.
- Pour in the beef stock.
- Add in the vinegar and bring to a boil. Simmer until slightly reduced, and season to taste.
- Add the mushrooms and cook until soft.
- Serve the rib roast with the ready-made balsamic-Portobello sauce.

RECIPE#40: STEAK ROLLS WITH BALSAMIC

Ingredients

- 1 1/2 – 2 lb. skirt steak, sliced thinly
- 1 carrot, (matchsticks)
- 1 bell pepper, (matchsticks)
- 1/2 a zucchini, (matchsticks)
- 6 green onions, (matchsticks)
- 2 cloves of garlic, minced
- 1/2 a teaspoon of dried oregano
- 1/2 a teaspoon of dried basil
- cooking fat
- salt and black pepper

Ingredients
Balsamic Glaze Sauce

- 1 tablespoon of ghee
- 2 tablespoons of shallots, finely chopped
- 1/4 of a cup of balsamic vinegar
- 1 tablespoon of organic honey
- 1/4 of a cup of beef stock
- salt and black pepper

Instructions

- Season the steak slices with salt and pepper to taste.
- Melt the ghee in a pan and place over a medium heat.
- Add the shallots and cook until soft, for about 2 minutes.
- Add the balsamic vinegar, organic honey, and the beef stock.
- Bring to a boil and simmer on low until the liquid is reduced by nearly half.
- Transfer to a bowl.
- In the same pan, add some cooking fat and cook the garlic for around 2 minutes, then add all the remaining vegetables and cook for about 3 to 4 minutes.
- Season with oregano, basil, and transfer into a bowl.
- Arrange vegetables in the center of each slice of beef.

Tightly rolling the meat around the filling and securing with wooden toothpicks.
- Return the beef rolls to the pan and cook over a medium heat.
- Remove the toothpicks and spoon balsamic sauce over the rolls.

RECIPE #41: STUFFED SWEET POTATO POCKETS

Ingredients
Toggle Units

- 1 lb. of ground beef
- 4 sweet potatoes
- 1/2 an onion, diced
- 1 tomato, diced
- 2 bell peppers, diced
- 1 cup of fresh lettuce, shredded
- 1/2 a cup of chopped green onions
- salsa

Ingredients
Taco Seasoning

- 1 tablespoon of chili powder
- 1 teaspoon of cumin (ground)
- 1/2 teaspoon of paprika (ground)
- 1/2 teaspoon of dried oregano
- 1/2 teaspoon of garlic powder
- salt and black pepper

Instructions

- Preheat your oven to 220 degrees Celsius.
- Pierce the potatoes with a fork and bake in the oven, directly on a rack, until soft for approx. 45 minutes.

- In a bowl, combine all the ingredients for the taco seasoning.
- Melt some cooking fat in a pan over a medium heat.
- Add the onions and cook until soft; about 4 minutes.
- Add the beef to the pan and cook until brown.
- Sprinkle the taco seasoning onto the beef and stir well.
- Cook the beef for another minute or two and then set aside.
- Slit each potato and push ends of each potato toward each other to open.
- Fill the potatoes with the beef and top with all of the remaining vegetables.
- Serve with your own homemade salsa.

RECIPE#42: BOLD AND BEAUTIFUL BEEF STEW

Ingredients

- 1lb. of beef cubes
- 1 butternut squash, peeled, de-seeded and diced
- 2 onions, diced
- 3 garlic cloves, minced
- 4 carrots, diced
- 6 oz. of mushrooms, sliced
- 6 oz. of spinach, chopped well
- 1 cup of chicken stock
- 14 oz. of diced tomatoes
- 1 tablespoon of chili powder
- 1 teaspoon of paprika
- 1 teaspoon of dried oregano
- salt and black pepper

Instructions

- Warm up a pan over a medium-high heat.
- Brown the beef in the pan for about 1 minute per side.
- Transfer the meat to a slow cooker.

- Add all remaining ingredients, except for the spinach and the mushrooms.
- Give everything a good stir and set the slow cooker to low and cook for 6 to 8 hours.
- Add in the mushrooms, about 30 minutes before the stew is completed.
- Add the spinach right before serving.

Chapter Six

PALEO SNACK RECIPES

Recipe#43: FETA (WITH ALMOND) CHEESE SPREAD

Ingredients

- 1 cup of almonds
- ¼ of a cup of lemon juice
- 3 tablespoons of olive oil
- 1/4 of a cup of olive oil
- 1 garlic clove
- 1 1/4 teaspoons of salt
- 1 tablespoon of thyme leaves
- 1 teaspoon of rosemary leaves

Instructions

- Place almonds in medium bowl and cover with 4 inches of water.
- Let them soak for 24 hours.
- Drain and rinse.
- Puree the almonds, lemon juice, the olive oil, garlic, salt and 1/2 a cup of water in blender for 6 minutes or until really creamy.

- Place a triple layer of cheesecloth into a strainer and spoon almond mixture onto it. Bring sides together twisting into an apple-sized ball and secure with a tie. Chill for 14 hours.
- Line baking sheet and transfer almond ball from cheesecloth. Shape into a 5" round of brie (about 3/4" thick).
- Bake for around 45 minutes.
- Cool. Then chill.
- Combine 1/4 of a cup of olive oil with herbs and heat over medium heat.
- Cool to room temperature and drop over almond spread just before serving.
- Spread onto crusty bread or crackers.

RECIPE#44: LUXURY LEMON SOUFFLE

Ingredients

- 1/2 of a cup of lemon juice
- 1 grated lemon rind
- 2 tablespoons of organic honey
- 3 eggs, separated
- ¾ of a cup of coconut milk

Instructions

- Preheat oven to 180 degrees Celsius, fan forced.
- In a bowl, mix together the lemon juice, lemon rind, honey, egg yolks (put the egg whites in a separate bowl) and the coconut milk.
- Beat the egg whites to form peaks.
- Now fold the peaked egg whites into the lemon mixture.
- Place mixture into 2 separate oven safe dishes, in an oven tray filled with water (to reach half way up).
- To help the soufflé rise evenly, run your finger around the edge of each dish.
- Bake in the oven for 25 minutes (approx.).

RECIPE#45: LOVELY TARTS WITH LEMON

Ingredients
Pastry

- 1 cup of almond meal
- 3 tablespoons of lemon juice
- 4 dates

Filling

- 6 tablespoons of lemon juice
- 1 lemon, rind grated
- 1 tablespoon of organic honey
- 2 eggs

Instructions

- Preheat oven to 180 degrees Celsius, fan -forced.
- To make the pastry, place ingredients into a blender and mix until combined.
- In a muffin tray, line individual holes with baking paper, and firmly place mixture on the bottom and sides.
- Bake in oven for 12 minutes. Leave to cool.
- To make the filling: place lemon juice, lemon rind and honey into a pan, and then simmer gently on low heat for 3 minutes.
- In a bowl, beat up the eggs well.
- Slowly add the beaten eggs to the simmering filling; stirring quickly to form a smooth texture. Leave to cool.
- When pastry has cooled, spoon the filling into each individual tart.
- Place in the fridge until cooled and set well.

RECIPE#46: LEMON AND RASPBERRY TARTS

Ingredients

- 1 cup of chopped walnuts
- 1 1/2 cups of almonds
- 1 1/2 cups dates

Filling

- 1 cup of coconut milk
- 1/3 of a cup of lemon juice
- 2 teaspoon of grated lemon rind
- 1 1/2 tablespoons of organic honey
- 8 eggs, beaten
- 2/3 of a cup of raspberries

Instructions

- Preheat oven to 180 degrees Celsius, fan-forced.
- Combine nuts and dates in a food processor. Place on high for 30-40 seconds for a coarser texture.
- Line a 25cm tart pan with baking paper.
- Press pastry evenly along the bottom and the sides. Now refrigerate while making the filling.
- To make filling: place the coconut milk, lemon juice, lemon rind and organic honey into a pan, and simmer on low heat for 3 minutes. Slowly add the (beaten) eggs to the simmering mixture, stirring quickly to form a smoother texture.
- Pour filling slowly into the pastry case.
- Bake in oven for 30 minutes.
- Top with raspberries.

RECIPE#47: FRUIT N' COCONUT CREAM

Ingredients

- ¼ of a cup of raw coconut milk
- 1 cup of mixed berries (seasonal)
- 1 cup of mangoes
- a pinch of grated coconut

Instructions

- Dice the mangoes slice the berries (choose seasonally) thinly.
- Place the compote of fruit into a bowl and drizzle the coconut cream over (as much as you require, to taste).
- This recipe is fantastic if you like or crave ice cream and you can also use duets of strawberries and blueberries, or other combinations of your choice.
- Sprinkle coconut flakes if you want to garnish.

RECIPE#48: APPLE BARS WITH COCONUT

Ingredients

- 1 cup of strawberries
- 2 cups of shredded apples
- 1 cup of shredded coconut
- 1/4 of a cup of melted coconut oil
- 1 tablespoon of honey

Instructions

- Ready the strawberries, and thaw if frozen.
- Melt down the coconut oil.
- Peel and shred the apples.

- Place all of the ingredients except for the coconut oil into the food processor.
- Pour the coconut oil over the coconut.
- Mix all of the ingredients together until all chunks are gone.
- Spread evenly onto a dehydrator pan, approximately a 1/4 inch thick.
- Dehydrate at 135°F for 5 hours.
- Cut into cubed portions and store in the refrigerator.

RECIPE#49: CRANBERRY-ORANGE BREAD

Ingredients

- 2 cups of fresh cranberries
- 4 eggs
- 1/4 cup and 1 tablespoon coconut oil, melted and divided
- 1/4 cup and 1 tablespoon of organic honey, divided
- 1/4 cup and 3 tablespoons of arrowroot powder, divided
- 1/4 cup and 2 tablespoons of coconut flour
- 2 teaspoons of baking powder
- the juice of two oranges
- the zest of one orange

Instructions

- Preheat the oven to 200 degrees Celsius.
- Grease a cake pan (8 or 9 inches) with coconut oil.
- Melt one tablespoon of coconut oil in a pan.
- In a bowl, mix one tablespoon of coconut oil, one tablespoon of arrowroot powder and one tablespoon of organic honey.
- Pour into the pan and distribute, spreading it evenly.
- Add cranberries on top of wet mixture. Spread evenly.
- In a separate bowl, mix the eggs, four tablespoons of coconut oil (melted), four tablespoons of organic honey, the

juice of one fresh orange and the zest of one fresh orange. Combine thoroughly.

- In a separate bowl, mix together the coconut flour, 1/4 cup and 2 tablespoons of the arrowroot powder, and the baking powder as well.
- Combine both the wet and dry ingredients into one bowl and mix really well.
- Pour combined mixture over cranberries, distributing evenly.
- Bake for 30 minutes.

RECIPE#50: COCONUT SPINACH WITH TANGY LEMON

Ingredients

- 2 teaspoons of oil
- 1 yellow onion
- 4 large cloves of garlic, minced
- 1 tablespoon of grated ginger
- 1/2 cup of sundried tomatoes, chopped
- 2 tablespoons of lemon juice
- 1/4 – 1/2 teaspoon of red pepper flakes
- 1 lb. of baby spinach
- a 14-ounce can of coconut milk
- 1 teaspoon of salt
- 1 teaspoon of ginger (ground)
- 2 breasts of cubed or shredded (cooked) chicken

Instructions

- Heat the oil in a large pot over medium-high heat.
- Add the onion and cook for about 6 minutes, or until the onion is brown.
- Add the garlic, ginger, sun-dried tomatoes, lemon zest and red pepper. Do this for 2-3 minutes, stirring frequently.

- Toss in the spinach, one small handful at a time. This will take about 6 minutes.
- When all the spinach has been gently added and stirred in, pour in the coconut milk and stir in the salt, ground ginger, and then the lemon juice.
- Add in cooked chicken and bring to a simmer.
- Now cook for 10 minutes or until the chicken is warmed through.

IN CONCLUSION

One night, my friend Jeremy came over for dinner (as he did most Saturday nights). Usually, we had some protein (like fish or chicken) combined with his least favorite... a salad of some kind.

That particular weekend, I made him a paleo casserole I'd learned from a chef on the TV. He was foaming at the mouth to eat it, and he said, "Oh, yay, it's not something and salad!" I laughed at his enthusiasm for the "yummy" food I was going to give him. At the time, I had a light-bulb moment... *the paleo really does allow you to eat well, and it tastes amazing!* In fact, I realized that you barely know you're on a diet! And that's such a winning point for me, and Jeremy. In truth, I got sick of salads too (although I never told Jeremy). I like to spoil him now, with great, yummy recipes.

So, I'm super-thrilled to say; that with the paleo I noticed a wonderful change. I felt good (and not desperately hungry like I had on other diet styles), and... I lost weight too! Yes, over 100 pounds. And my arthritis inflammation was also diminished; to the point of barely any pain. My mother also learned many of the recipes with me, and we enjoyed the time we spent together in the kitchen, so that was a big plus, too.

I guess for me, using the paleo is easy. The rules, the foods, and the flavors of real, wholesome, yummy foods. That's what makes it awesome for me. I know that if you're trying to lose weight, and you want to do it healthily, the paleo is something that's a real blessing in disguise. I truly hope you love the recipes you find here. I have made every one of them.

So, we made it!! Oh yes, that was awesome wasn't it? I really hope so, because it has worked for me... so very well. In conclusion, I want to say a huge thank you to you again, for caring about yourself enough to keep going on this wonderful journey!

Every recipe in this book is tried and tested by me and all of them can be tweaked to suit your tastes. So, add a bit more pepper, or make double the marinade and freeze some for next time if you want! You are the boss in your kitchen.

If you can, a great idea is to make 4 recipes over a weekend and then you can use them during the week, if you freeze them. I know this is awesome, because I did it loads of times, and if you work during the week you can sometimes be far too tired to cook when you get home from work. That's for sure!

I ask you to believe in yourself as much as you can. I want you to know how magnificent you are. And once you set your mind on it, the world is (metaphorically) your oyster... that's a fun diet joke, by the way! So, I wish you a happy and a healthy weight loss journey, and I thank you for being with me here. I know you've got this! Yes, you totally do.

So, I am sending you all of my love and best wishes for the future,

Lots of love and light always, *Emma xx*

P.S. Oh, don't forget; if you haven't already read my title, "How I Lost 100 Pounds! My Personal Weight Loss Strategies for Optimum Happiness," make sure you get your FREE copy today. Inside you'll learn exactly how I lost my weight, and the benefits of knowing the must-do nutrition, and other amazing secrets including myths, water weight, cellulite prevention and removal, the only exercise you really need, the ancient and easy technique to help slim you quickly, how to balance meals, and much, much more! I hope you love it. It's my amazing gift to you! You rock!!

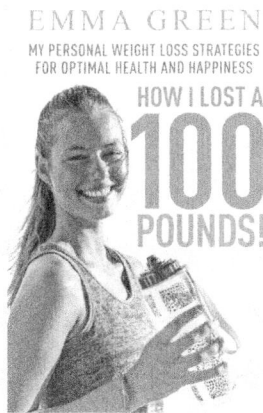

EMMA GREEN
MY PERSONAL WEIGHT LOSS STRATEGIES
FOR OPTIMAL HEALTH AND HAPPINESS
HOW I LOST A
100
POUNDS!

Click here to get your FREE copy or check out my profile for other free titles

Printed in Great Britain
by Amazon

18638241R00041